The Silhouette Solution

Lose The Weight You Want And
Have The Silhouette You Choose

David Macallan, N.M.D.

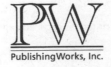
PublishingWorks, Inc.

PublishingWorks, Inc.,
151 Epping Road
Exeter, NH 03833
603-778-9883

For Sales and Orders:
800-768-7667

LCCN: 2008941371
ISBN: 1-933002-75-1
ISBN-13: 978-1-933002-75-0

Printed on recycled paper.

Printed in Canada.

The Silhouette Solution

Acknowledgments

Producing even a simple little book like this is an enormous undertaking, involving countless people besides the author. Tim Gilbert did a magnificent job on the cover, Tom Bartoloni laid out the book and made sure it was ready for publication, and Denise Autry, RN, CCN and Eliot Bolan, BS, MS, MBA provided expert technical review.

I must acknowledge Professor Albert Stunkard, who I know only by reputation, for his original research using silhouettes to assess weight – although we used our own silhouettes for this publication. Professor George Blackburn's work on the Set Point proved invaluable in helping explain how people can maintain weight loss long term.

My naturopathic physician colleagues might have expected me to produce a scholarly text, rather than this little story, yet the message it contains reflects the work of dozens of my colleagues and teachers. I humbly acknowledge their dedicated practice and scholarship.

There are many non-profit organizations whose mission is to help consumers understand the importance of good nutrition, and I acknowledge the difficult work they do tackling the "enemy at the gate."

A handful of companies now specialize in designing and producing carefully calibrated food, both for weight loss and weight maintenance. I thank them for making it easy for people to lose weight simply as they learn to recalibrate their own food intake.

Todd Stanwood, Scott Stanwood and Lou DiCaprio provided me with the opportunity to touch thousands of lives with the work I do for them. They were kind enough to allow me to disappear from the office for days at a time to complete this book. Thanks in particular to mastermind mentor Todd for driving this book to publication in record time.

Samantha Davis was kind enough to remain patient with me at home as I remained glued to my screen for countless hours.

Finally, I acknowledge all of you, my readers. You can use this book the change lives for the better. Spread the word.

Table of Contents

Introduction

One day I looked in the mirror and saw someone I barely recognized. I knew I'd been gaining weight, but that day I just *looked* different. Maybe that final pound was simply the last straw. I knew it had to stop.

That was the day I became obese. It seems like an abstract line in the sand, but crossing the obesity line comes with a laundry list of consequences. Being overweight has its own troubles, but obesity multiplies your risk of developing a slew of diseases. You'd have thought a nutritional doctor like me would have known better. When I went to medical school I was 32 years old and 140 pounds. Yet in what seemed like the blink of an eye I was 53 and weighed 217.

My weight just kept creeping up. I couldn't seem to stop it, even though I was getting plenty of exercise. I vowed that when it got over 180 I would absolutely have to do something about it; but I didn't. It passed 190 and still I did nothing. When 200 came and went, I numbly wondered how a weight that at one time was unimaginably far in the distance in front of me could now be far behind in the rear view mirror. And still it climbed.

Being overweight was no fun, but I tolerated it for a while, and compensated heavily. I did some of the things you've probably done: wore only black or navy to keep me looking thinner; wore shirts over my pants instead of tucking them in; bought blousy shirts, nothing contouring; wore jackets or a flattering sport coat everywhere; kept them buttoned so no-one could see the blubber above the beltline; never went in a swimming pool or sauna;

just kept out of situations that required anyone to see what lay beneath my protective clothing. At some point, I even accepted it, and the little voice inside told me that since I wasn't doing anything about it, I might as well keep eating. Many people have told me they've heard that same little voice.

You may think I should have known better, and you would be right. I've been passionate about nutrition for nearly 30 years, and I've seen the dramatic benefits people enjoy when they get the nutritional part of their lives right. Many of them were my patients. Yet for some reason, during a few years of ferocious stress, I didn't seem able to apply those countless hours of education and practice on myself. I just wanted to eat. And that gives us a clue about what's going on in this country. If I, with full professional knowledge of nutrition, ended up nearly 50 pounds overweight, how difficult must it be for the majority of people who have no special knowledge to maintain a healthy weight?

That's when I resolved to take care of my own weight problem, and while I was doing it, figure out how to help you do the same. I have succeeded in dropping my excess weight, and so can you. That's what this book is about. *Your* weight loss success. Since I've learned that people remember stories better than they remember cold, hard facts, what follows is a story whose characters are based on people I've met along the way. And while the facts sprinkled through the book are powerful, what's more important is that you get shocked, angry, inspired, passionate and committed to your success.

Yours in health,

Dr. Mac

Prologue

The wedding preparations were in full swing, but Paul was restless. He kept trying to think of tasks to keep him occupied, but found himself pacing anxiously up and down the yard. His twin brother Steve, whom he hadn't seen in five years, was due at any moment. Steve's first overseas assignment was meant to be for two years – and that would have been long enough for Paul. But one responsibility had led to another, and now it had been five.

"There's just too much going on," Steve would always say. "I can't get away. I'm halfway around the world – and it takes me at least two days each way. I'll come next year." It was their sister's wedding that finally brought Steve home.

It wasn't as though they hadn't spoken. They'd kept in touch by phone every other week, but it was mostly e-mail, with the usual jokes, jibes, cartoons, little stories and seasonal greetings shuttling back and forth that had kept the connection.

Born within minutes of each other, they'd remained together for much of the ensuing 35 years, until Steve's work forced them apart. As kids and teenagers they'd loved to play the kinds of pranks that only identical twins can – and now they'd get to again because Paul had some new people in his circle that hadn't met Steve. He'd carefully assembled some matching outfits that would do the trick. Paul grinned as he thought of the pranks they could once again play now that he had his sparring partner back.

A familiar yell startled him back to his senses.

"Pauleeee!" Steve bellowed as he hauled himself out of the taxi. "What's up?"

Paul whirled around and took off down the yard. "Steve-O!" he yelled back as he ran to greet his brother. Paul's step faltered a little as he caught sight of Steve, or who he thought was Steve. The visitor sounded like his brother but didn't look like him.

"Wow", he thought to himself. "What happened? I know that's got to be him, but man, he's gotten big. He's got a moon face."

Paul caught himself quickly. "No weight discrimination allowed here," he thought. "Oh, well, maybe a little . . . just for fun . . . it's Steve, after all . . ."

Paul and Steve hugged and slapped each other on the back, punched the air, gave each other high-fives and did some whooping and hollering.

"Welcome home!" said Paul. "It's just great to see you again."

"Back atcha, bro. I've missed this place," said Steve, taking in the familiar landscape.

"And hey," Paul whacked Steve on the stomach. "You never told me you were pregnant. Who's the lucky lady?"

He expected a quick rebuttal, but instead Steve's face fell. "Man, much as I've been looking forward to this moment, I've been dreading it too," he said. "I knew I'd be taking some serious ribbing from everyone about my weight, and here we go, right out of the gate. You know what, Pauley? I thought twice about coming back at all, and that's really why I haven't been home. I wanted to get it handled first," he added, "but I didn't have any control over when sis got married. So here I am, and I just don't want to hear one more word about my weight, OK?"

"Oh man", thought Paul, that wasn't the best start!" He put his arm around his brother as they walked towards the house. "Hey Steve," he said, keeping his voice down. "I'm sorry. It's been a while and you never said anything about it and I had no idea it was such a tender spot. Not one more word, I promise." Paul raised his voice. "Let's just move on and join the gang. Everybody's thrilled you're here."

"Hey sir?" yelled the cab driver. "Do you want your luggage?" Steve thumped his forehead with his palm. "Aw gee, I'd forget my head if it wasn't screwed on," and trotted off to get his suitcase.

Paul grabbed his chance and raced into the house. "Listen up quickly, everyone. Steve just got here, and there's a lot more of him than there was before. He's super sensitive about it – so not one word, OK?"

"OK," they all nodded from around the breakfast bar, "not a word." Paul dashed back out of the house to grab the suitcase from Steve as he paid the driver. "Boy," he thought, "That was a close call but I think we got away with it."

As they strolled back up the path, Steve looked quizzically at his brother. "Hey, how come you got skinny while I was working on doubling up? We're identical twins with exactly the same genes. When I left 5 years ago, we were both about twenty pounds over, and now here I am at 240 and you're at what? 180? Less?"

"Less," said Paul. "I'm at 173, which is right about where a five foot ten guy needs to be. But you said you didn't want to talk about it any more!"

"That's right," Steve shot back. "I don't want to talk about my weight *gain*. But I do want to talk about your weight *loss* because if we have the same body, and I do what you did, I'll get the same results, right?"

"Well, I'm not a doctor, but I figure you would," Paul replied as they walked up to the porch. "Because like you, I packed on some more after you left, but I was able to knock it off easily once I understood what was going on. Sure, I had a few false starts, but I've gotten the hang of it now, and there are only six things you need to know."

"That's the best news I've heard in a long time. Just don't tell me I'm going to have to eat celery all day," Steve retorted, with a loud guffaw. "No rabbit food for Steve."

"No worries, man," Paul replied. "I seem like I'm never done eating."

"That sounds more like it," said Steve with a grin. "And talking of eating, let's see what they've put out on the breakfast bar. I could eat a horse after a flight with nothing but peanuts."

Chapter One: Enemy at the Gates

"Man, that was good," exclaimed Steve as he pushed his chair back from the table and patted his belly. "Lots of the treats I like. I love family parties."

"Yeah bro, no kidding," agreed Paul. "There's nothing to beat that good old home cooking, just like when we were growing up. And it never tastes right unless mom makes it."

"Yeah, I've really missed this," said Steve, waving his hand at the spread before them. "But help me understand one thing, Pauley. If we like the same stuff, how come you ended up like you and I ended up like me?"

"Well, you're here for a month, and I said there were only six things you needed to know, so if we just make sure we get a little time together, between all the other folks who want to visit with you, I can tell my story and maybe some of it will help," replied Paul. "Once you understand what to do, it's pretty simple… and there's no-one I'd love to help more than you. We need to be able to get up to our old tricks again. So I need my body twin back."

"Now wait a minute, P-man," Steve interjected. "Answer one question for me. You told me you'd packed on a bunch of weight after I left, so we really could have <u>stayed</u> body doubles, just bigger. Tell me, how big did you get?"

Paul winced as he thought back. "Truthfully, I wasn't that far behind you. I ate myself all the way up to 220 pounds. Felt terrible, tried a few things, but even if I dropped a few pounds, they always came right back on. I just don't like starving and it always seemed that diets were to do with <u>not</u> eating."

He waved around the room. "Just look around you. We grew up in a family that loves to eat. It's a big social thing as well as a taste thing, so not eating was not an option for me."

"Hallelujah," sang Steve. "Gimme food!" They both laughed loud and hard and clinked their glasses in a toast. "To food, food and more food."

"OK bro," said Steve, getting suddenly serious. "Fess up. Howd'ya get it done?"

"Roll into the living room… Oops, sorry. Follow me in there and I'll tell you. I don't want to be tempted by all these desserts," Paul said as he headed through the door. "Let's get our feet up while everyone else is busy in the kitchen."

Paul settled into the couch and put his feet on an ottoman. "Man, that's as much as I've eaten in a long time."

"Yeah, me too," responded Steve as he fell back into a recliner opposite Paul. "I'm so stuffed I'll need a winch to get back up."

Paul leaned back in the couch. "OK, Steve, here's how it went. I was in a really lousy mood one day, not feeling good, low energy, clothes feeling too tight, and I go in for my routine checkup. The doc says I've now gained enough weight to be called obese. My blood pressure is way up, my cholesterol's high, I'm within a hair of having diabetes, and the extra weight has been trashing my knees. His solution was four drug prescriptions and a stern order for me to lose weight. He said it was nobody's fault but my own and if I ate less I might drop some poundage and get off the prescriptions. Otherwise I'd be on them for life."

"You mean like the four prescriptions *I'm* on?" Steve interjected. "Funny how that works."

"Well funny, but not really," Paul retorted. "So I asked if he had any advice about that and he just told me to eat less. To keep eating what I was already eating, but leave half of it on the plate. He said anybody could do it."

"Well, I was fuming by the time I left his office. A fat lot of help *that* was. And the worst of it was, the doc was overweight himself. But I resolved right there and then I was gonna show him!"

"So let me ask you something, Stevie. How long do you think I lasted?"

"Tell me," asked Steve.

"A day," Paul admitted sheepishly.

"A day?" Steve guffawed from his chair. "If it was me, I might have managed one *meal*." "Naw," he added, shaking his head. "Not even that."

"Exactly," Paul responded, shaking his pointed finger repeatedly at the kitchen. "You remember how we were brought up, right? Whatever's on your plate . . ."

"Yep," Steve completed the sentence. "You finish."

"That's right," Paul went on. "You finish your plate. So I did. And figuring out how to put only half on the plate was tough too. Most of the time I'm not doing it. Someone else is. Either here at home or in a restaurant. And here's the other thing. If I did eat a half portion, I was ravenous within twenty minutes. I went back and ate the rest. It just didn't work."

"I'm not surprised," Steve chimed in. "Wouldn't have worked for me either."

"But I was damned if I was going to let that doc get the better of me," said Paul. "I still had a head of steam going when I got back to the office, and I wasn't exactly being quiet about it. So one of the other journalists told me he'd just done a story with a nutritional doctor and maybe I should talk to her. I figured, hey, I'm going to treat this like a news story. I'm going to do an investigation, and I'm going to get this weight thing figured out. I'm going to get to the bottom of it."

"And by the way, Steve, your engineer's mind will find some of this story very interesting . . ."

– – – – – –

A water sculpture tinkled gently in the waiting room as Paul checked in for his appointment. Large, brightly colored tropical fish meandered around in an aquarium as other smaller ones darted from one end of the tank to the other. As Paul marveled at a boxy blowfish, the door behind him opened and an attractive woman in a white coat walked purposefully towards him, hand outstretched. Her stethoscope swung as she walked. "Hi, Paul, I'm Dr. Wendy. Nice to meet you. Come on back."

"Pleased to meet you too," he replied, matching her pace into the corridor. "Wow," he said, waving at a room they passed. "That's quite a pharmacy you've got there!"

"Yes," she said. "It's tough to get medical-grade nutritional products in stores, so we dispense them here."

"I didn't know there was such a thing as a medical-grade supplement."

"Oh, I'm sure you'll know all about them soon enough," she said over her shoulder. Take a seat, and I'll be with you in a moment."

"Thanks," Paul nodded, using the opportunity to take a good look around the room. Books lined the shelves behind her desk: biochemistry, nutrition, anatomy, pathology, physiology, microbiology, minor surgery, herbal medicine, a stack of journals. "Hmmmm, that's interesting," he thought. "A whole section on PR, branding, demographics… she must be trying to market herself."

On the wall beside her desk, several diplomas hung neatly. Paul walked over for a closer look. "Doctor of Naturopathic Medicine, 1991. A state license. A voluntary service award. So far, so good.

"Checking me out, are you?" Wendy laughed as she walked back in.

"Darn right I was," he responded quickly, as they both settled into matching chairs opposite her desk. "I haven't been to a naturopathic physician before. I see all your diplomas, but what kind of training did you have?"

"A lot", replied Wendy. "Four years pre-med, four years postgraduate, just like regular doctors, but instead of focusing on hospital work, we do all our training in out-patient offices, and focus on nutrition, botanicals, physical medicine and lots of other areas. That's why people come to see us."

"Interesting stuff," remarked Paul. "So do you 'say no to drugs?'"

"Oh, I can write prescriptions," she said with a smile. "And they're important from time to time, but I'd hate it if prescribing was the only tool I had."

"Now *that* one I understand," said Paul. "Reminds me of the old phrase 'If the only tool you've got is a hammer, everything looks like a nail'."

"You got it," nodded Wendy with a laugh. "So anyway, my mission is to help you with your health, and we do indeed have a lot of tools for that. So how can I help you?"

"Well, my doctor told me I needed to lose weight, but he wasn't much help with the 'how', Paul started in. "He said I was just eating too much and needed to cut back; that it was just my fault for not being able to control myself. I think there's probably more to it than that."

"No doubt about it," Wendy exclaimed. "And let me start by taking the guilt off your shoulders right now." She looked at Paul squarely. "It is, for the most part, *not your fault*."

"Not my fault?" said Paul, a little surprised. "But I'm the one that puts the food in my mouth. How can it not be my fault?"

"It's really simple," Wendy replied. "You're thinking you're the cause, but you're really the effect." She turned and waved at the shelves of books he'd looked at earlier. "It's all in there, and it took years for scientists to put it together. And you need to understand marketing, too. But let me give you the simple version. It's not just something you did. It's also something that was done *to* you."

"Doctor," Paul interjected. "I'm an adult, I make my own choices. Plus, I'm a journalist, so I've seen it all and I'm not easily manipulated."

"Exactly," said Wendy, picking up the pace. "And that's the way most people feel, and that's why they become prey."

"Prey? I never felt like prey, except at a car dealership or a furniture store," Paul joked.

Wendy didn't hesitate for a moment. "I totally understand. And as soon as you get the hang of this, you'll have taken the first step towards changing its effect on your life. Will you stay with me on this?"

The cynic in Paul, born of years of journalism, started to rebel. He hadn't expected the conversation to go this way, but OK, he thought, he'd listen . . . this was an investigation after all . . .

"People always justify the choices they make. It's how they stay feeling good about themselves and the things they're doing, right?" Wendy continued.

"All right, I'll buy that," he replied. "I've seen it often enough in my professional life."

Wendy pressed on. "So what if I told you that *billions* of dollars are spent each year convincing, manipulating, even seducing you into making some or all of the choices for your health, right or wrong, which you then justify as being OK?"

"Hmmmm, I'm staying with you for the moment," Paul said. "Go on."

"It's orchestrated by some of the smartest, brightest, most highly paid people in the country," Wendy continued.

"Madison Avenue, right?" Paul suggested. "I'm no stranger to advertisers and they sure know how to push people's buttons."

Wendy set her clipboard on her lap and leaned forward in her chair. "So far so good, but are you ready for the part most people are completely unaware of?"

"I'm all ears," he responded, leaning forward and matching Wendy's gaze . . .

"What if I told you that the food and beverage companies paying the advertisers are well aware that many of the foods they are promoting will inevitably make you fat?"

"All right. So if you eat more, you're going to gain weight. No surprise there, Doc." That was pretty obvious, he thought.

Then Wendy threw the curve ball. "Would it make any difference to your thinking if I told you they know they are making you fat, but some don't want to change the products and marketing they've developed and used over the last century?"

"Wow," Paul said, jerking his head back in surprise. "It's hard for me to accept that companies wouldn't be all over this. Don't they have any social conscience?"

"Well, some do and some don't," Wendy replied emphatically. "Some food companies are making an effort to create more wholesome, natural foods. But, unfortunately, far too many companies are still driven solely to make their shareholders happy. These companies are actually delighted to discover that the products they've been promoting are not only cheap to make and profitable, but are addicting to the human body."

Paul was reeling. "Well I guess that's one way to think about it," he said. "But it sounds like you're one of those conspiracy theorists."

Wendy chuckled. "Not at all. It all started perfectly naturally, and all the parts were independent. Nobody planned it. It just got twisted and messed up along the way. And now much of it is planned."

"OK, so if I'm going to believe you, Dr. Wendy," said Paul, "you're going to have to convince me that what they do is addictive and they know it."

"Hey, I'm happy to," Wendy shot right back. "Because once you see how all the parts fit together as I unravel them for you, two things will happen. First, you'll get angry and want to fight back, and second, you'll understand what to do about it in the long run. The first will get you skinnier quite naturally. The second will keep you that way for life."

"I'm ready," said Paul as he pulled out his notepad. "Shoot."

"Remember how I said it was simple and complicated at the same time?" Wendy started out.

Paul nodded his head: "Yep, I remember."

"So," she continued. "I could spend time talking about a bunch of things-- the change from what we all ate a few hundred years ago compared to now, or the shift from agriculture into agribusiness, the industrialization of the food supply, the addition of chemicals, the huge increase in additives; or, as I call them, just by adding a 'c': 'addictives'. But, to your great relief, I'm sure, I'm going to focus on only one thing here since I've already talked about advertising," she added. "And it's this: carbohydrates, sugars, and a condition called insulin resistance that many people in this country suffer from."

"Carbohydrates I have heard lots about, but not so much about insulin resistance," said Paul, with a quizzical smile on his face. "I guess I'm about to become an expert."

Wendy smiled. "No need to become an expert, but everyone who understands the basics of this gets to live in a different world from everyone else. They get to experience a new sense of freedom, if they want."

"It all sounds good to me," Paul said. "How simple can you make it?"

"Really simple," she said. "And once you get it, well, I'm not saying you'll never be fooled again, but it will be way harder, because you'll see them coming . . ."

This is pretty intriguing, thought Paul. "And a different kind of doctor visit. What was this 'hidden knowledge' Dr. Wendy was talking about?

"It is so simple, but so profound," she began, then turned to Paul and asked, "Not that long ago, when we humans were making the best of what was around us, what did we eat?"

"Well, it's hard for me to visualize that," he admitted. "But it seems from some TV shows I've seen that even a few hundred years ago, we were all eating meat, mostly hunted on the hoof, fresh and seawater fish, lots of vegetables, fruit in season, maybe some grains, but not a whole lot else, except maybe insects in some places. Am I close?"

"Very close." Wendy replied. "And by the way, the human body works best with that kind of combination. That's how the body's calibrated. Are you familiar with the concept of calibration?"

"Yes, I've reported on a few things where calibration comes into play," replied Paul, looking off to the side as he reached back into memory. "Let's see. It was usually about equipment, and making sure the settings were right, so it would do what it was meant to do . . ."

"And if the equipment was not calibrated properly?" asked Wendy.

"OK," Paul continued. "Then there would be all kinds of problems. Like if a thermostat isn't calibrated properly, a room will get too hot or too cold. Or if a car's fuel system isn't calibrated properly then it will run rough, or spew nasty exhaust fumes."

"Precisely," said Wendy. "Now here's the trick. With the thermostat and the car engine, you adjust *them* to alter the fuel flow. But the body is the *total opposite*. The settings are hard-wired genetically and you can't change them. In other words, the calibration's fixed. And because you can't recalibrate the body, you have to calibrate the fuel."

"Wow, I see where you're going with this," said Paul. "So you're saying that the body's just doing what it's designed to do, and we can't change that. Therefore we have to *calibrate the food to the body because we can't do it the other way around*."

"Yes, it's as simple as that" Wendy agreed. "And most of the commercially prepared food out there is not properly calibrated for the human body. That's why it wreaks so much havoc on people's weight, cholesterol levels, blood pressure and on and on."

"Yet people just keep eating it," mused Paul. "Just like smokers keep smoking and drinkers keep drinking, even though it's slowly killing them, me included."

"It's much more profound than just 'eat better'," Wendy continued. "And it's most obvious with sugars – carbs, as most people call them now. The food companies scored a lucky slam-dunk with that one."

"How'd you mean *lucky*?" Paul interjected; "Didn't you just say this whole thing was intentional on the part of some food companies?"

"Well it is now, but it didn't start out that way," said Wendy. "It simply started out as a way to make more money, and there's nothing wrong with that. People had been eating grains in one form or another for a long time. But they were always whole grains and the people eating them were in motion all day long, not like today."

Paul threw his hands in the air. "No kidding. I used to exercise all the time, but now there never seem to be enough hours in the day."

"Right, but I'm not even talking about exercise in that way. I'm talking about people having intensely physical lives. It's only recently that we've all become sedentary and even had to *think* about exercise. But we'll get to that later. Right now, I want you to understand *this*." Wendy pointed at a diagram on the wall. "This is human metabolism. It shows how all the body's chemicals work together – how it's calibrated. That part on the left is sugar metabolism."

"Yikes, that looks like a map of LA, and it would take me a long time to find my way around. Go easy on me," joked Paul.

"Don't worry, you don't need to know any detail, just one simple fact," Wendy went on. "Complex carbs, like those found in whole grains, raise blood sugar very slowly. That's how blood sugar is meant to work."

"But even as long ago as the time of the Roman Empire, millers discovered how to separate out the two parts of the wheat to make white, starchy flour. They found that people would pay *more* for bread made out of white flour. And although they didn't know it back then, the brown bran was the best part, containing fiber, oils, vitamins and minerals."

"Entrepreneurship at work, eh?" commented Paul.

Wendy shrugged her shoulders and looked around the room. "Well, I have no objection to business. After all, I run a business here. But in the case of the millers, their neat business idea had devastating consequences that affect us all today – and it is one of the main causes of your weight problem."

"Oh, it's the *Romans* fault," Paul joked. "I should have known – those darn millers. How did that one thing have such a huge impact?"

"Two reasons: First, it threw *that* completely out of whack." Wendy pointed again at the metabolic map. "And second, it marked the beginning of refining, or food processing as we know it today. It didn't become a huge problem until the Industrial Revolution made white bread and other refined carbs like sugar affordable for everybody. Eventually, they fortified the flour with vitamins and minerals, thinking that would take care of it. But that was long before scientists realized the other devastating effect of refined grains on the human body – blood sugar and insulin spikes."

Wendy could see the interest growing on Paul's face, so she carried on. "When simple carbs get into the body, they spike the blood sugar very fast, and force the body to compensate just as fast. People get a burst of energy, then crash. And what do they do then?"

"Oh, I see where you're going with this," said Paul with an "aha" look on his face. "They reach for more. I do that myself all the time. I have cereal for breakfast and feel fine for a while, but next thing I know I'm flagging and I reach for a muffin."

"Righhhhhhhht." Wendy cocked her head and grinned. "And do you know what happens every time you go through that cycle? All the carbs that aren't used are converted to fat."

"Fat?" exclaimed Paul. "I thought it was fat that made fat. Isn't that why people are told to eat a low-fat diet?"

"No, it's not always the fat. It *can* be, but do you remember when we were told we should be eating less fat and eating bread and pasta?" Wendy asked.

Paul looked as though someone had turned a light on. "Oh yes, I remember that well. My mom did it and she packed on about 20 pounds. She complained that her cholesterol got worse too. It seemed like it had the opposite effect than it was meant to."

"Yes", Wendy agreed. "And she wasn't the only one. Since those days the US population has become the fattest on Earth. Three out of every four people are overweight and half of those are obese. It costs billions of dollars of taxpayers' money to treat all the diseases that result from this, while at the same time, it's been a bonanza for many of the food companies."

"Wow, this is wild!" said Paul, shaking his head. "But why hasn't it changed, now that we know?"

Wendy picked up the pace. "Good point," she said. "It goes back to what I said before. Some companies are trying to make healthier products, but many continue to delight in their 'metabolically addictive' cheap refined ingredients. So they keep designing more products with these ultra-cheap ingredients of refined flour, fat, sugar and salt, and to make them palatable, they concoct them into different textures and use a ton of chemicals to make them addictively tasty. People get hooked and some food companies in turn get hooked on the profits they're making. So whatever the consequences for people's health, they keep doing it . . ."

She said the last four words one at a time, giving them special emphasis, then fell silent, to let it sink in.

"Well, well, well," said Paul after a while. "I guess at you're saying that most packaged foods are not properly calibrated."

Wendy looked up. "They're not properly calibrated for the human body, but many are perfectly calibrated for the corporate bottom line. Just think about it: ultra-cheap ingredients, addictive characteristics, repeat buying and people don't even know. They think the way they feel is normal, but it's not, it's engineered."

"So this affects how people feel, too?" Paul asked, leaning forward in his chair.

"Oh yes, big time." Wendy waved her hand in the direction of the waiting room. "Let me give you an example. You were looking at the fish in the aquarium. Do you think they're aware that they're in water?"

Paul's brow furrowed. "I really have no idea, but I guess they would, right? That's where they live."

"Well, let's go with that for the moment." Wendy looked mischievously at Paul over the top of her spectacles. "And if they get out of the water?"

"Easy," Paul replied. "They're going to notice right away – and not in a good way."

"But when people get out of the soup, they notice it within days, and in a *good* way . . ." Wendy began.

"Soup? What soup?" Paul interjected.

"The soup of messed-up metabolism: food addictions they don't know they have, tens of thousands of advertising impressions every day, the illusion that cheap foods are actually valuable when they're made for cents on the dollar, stimulant drinks loaded with sugar and alcohol loaded with calories. *That* soup!"

Wendy thumped her clipboard emphatically on her knees. "Just like the fish, people don't even know they're in it until they get out of it. But in the case of people, once they get out of the soup, they feel like a million bucks. And they all tell me they feel a wonderful sense of freedom."

"Ouch," said Paul, after a while. "What you're saying makes total sense. But how come this is the first I've heard of it? Why isn't it talked about more? As a journalist, I thought I understood things pretty well, but this all seems worthy of a front page story."

Wendy shrugged her shoulders. "It's been tried, but it doesn't stick for long. There's just too much profit in keeping everyone's nose in the trough. And advertising dollars control the media. When was the last time you saw an ad for broccoli?"

"Broccoli?" laughed Paul, "Never."

"And why is that?" Wendy inquired with quizzical look.

It was starting to make sense to Paul. "I guess because there's not enough profit in it to pay for the ads."

"Bingo!" exclaimed Wendy, handing him a pad of paper. "You can be certain that you're overpaying for any food you see advertised on TV because the ingredients have to be cheap enough to allow for a marketing budget. It's business 101. And the cheapest ingredients . . ."

Paul jumped in and finished the sentence. ". . . are the ones that make us fat. People just don't think this through, do they?"

"No, they don't," said Wendy, shaking her head. "That's why it's a shared responsibility. Nothing will change until we stop putting that stuff in our mouths, force them to make better products by buying selectively and vote with our dollars. That'll make them sit up and take notice."

"Can't the government do anything about it?" asked Paul with a puzzled look.

"Well, there are guidelines out there, and non-profits that make some noise about it," Wendy shrugged, "but it's the big bucks that can shout the loudest."

She looked over at Paul. "So that brings us to you. Is this making sense so far?"

"It sure is." He replied. "I can see why you said it was simple and complicated. It's all interwoven in our society. But do you have a solution for me?"

"I do," she smiled. "I do. There only six things you need to know to normalize your weight for life, and here's the first. Jot this down…

'Enemy At The Gates'.

And remember as you start your weight loss that you're surrounded by marketing messages on TV, radio, in print, on billboards, and they're going to want your dollars. You've also got an enemy inside – the little voice that will try to derail you as your body changes."

"Just pin this statement somewhere you'll see it every day, and keep saying it out loud to yourself," Wendy said emphatically. "It'll keep you alert."

A note to myself

Chapter 1:
Enemy at the Gate

A different kind of doctor
It's not all my fault
Don't believe the ads
Knowledge is power
Carbs have consequences
Leave mis-calibrated foods alone
Break free

Chapter Two:
State Your Goals

The effects of lunch had hit full force and Steve was sprawled back on the recliner looking like he was ready to nod off.

"Steve-O!" yelled Paul from the sofa, knowing he needed to rouse his brother. "Step into my office and let me show you how I got started." He eased himself up. "The first part was really simple, so let's see if it makes as much sense to you as it did to me."

"OK," said Steve. "I'm heading your way, but let me just swing by the kitchen and pick up a dessert first."

Not even a minute later Steve strolled nonchalantly into Paul's office holding a big plate of cheesecake and ice cream, and making appreciative sounds. He stopped in his tracks when he saw what Paul was holding up.

"What in the world are those?" he asked.

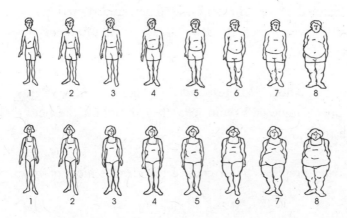

"Silhouettes, that's what," Paul responded. "During my first visit with Dr. Wendy, she asked me to pick which one of these I was and I picked number six. Where do you think you are on the scale?"

"Oh man, oh man," said Steve. "You said I looked pregnant so maybe I'm off the scale altogether!"

Paul sensed Steve's humor was an attempt to conceal some resistance, so he jumped back in. "Aw, come on, be a sport. Seriously, which silhouette do you think you are?"

Steve bobbed his head back and forth like some kind of strange exotic bird, examining the chart closely. "Well I guess I'd have to say number seven."

"OK great," said Paul. "So here's what Dr. Wendy said to me. As we age, we tend to move from left to right unless we're carefully watching what we eat, and that's what you and I *both* did. We were silhouette four in our twenties, then we both went up to number six."

"Yeah, yeah, yeah, and I won because I got to seven before you", exclaimed Steve. "But help me understand something … because I know you were the same … why is all my weight on my belly?"

"Aha, good question," Paul responded. "Remember how Wendy talked about simple carbs and how they throw off the body's metabolism?

"Yep . . . Steve replied. "How could I forget? It's most of what I eat."

"Hey, let's stay serious here," said Paul. "It's as simple as this. People who just plain eat too much gain weight all over; people who have hormonal weight gain, especially women, will tend to pack it on around the hips and thighs, like a pear shape. But people who have issues metabolizing carbs will pack the weight on around the middle, like an apple shape."

"Well," said Steve. "I've got some of the first one, but mostly the last one. So what?"

Paul shook his head. "Ahh, Steve-O, you're going to wish you hadn't asked. Let me ask you something. Is your belly still hard?"

Steve thumped on his belly. "Yeah, it is – and that's why I know I'm not as fat as I look. I'm big – but there's barely an inch or two of fat over my stomach muscles."

"I hear you, Steve," Paul responded. "And that's what I thought too – but it's because there was something I didn't know . . . and obviously you don't either."

Steve slumped in his chair. "Oh boy, what am I missing?"

Paul looked Steve squarely in the eye. "This may be the most important thing you've ever heard, so listen up. It turns out that the fat created by overeating, especially from too many carbs, doesn't just show up outside the stomach muscles. It builds *inside*, underneath the muscles!"

"Eeooooooow!" said Steve, thumping his belly again. "So I've got something inside? Like that movie when the alien was in there?"

"Funny you should use that term. That's exactly what Wendy called mine. Yep, it's a thing called the omentum, a chunk of fatty tissue that sits in front of your internal organs and wraps around some of them. It should be small, but overweight people, especially with carb issues, tend to grow one that's big," Paul continued.

"Does it do any damage inside?" interrupted Steve, suddenly visibly worried.

Paul knew his twin was having the same issues he'd had. "Yes, that's the problem, bro, the fat in the abdomen is not storage. It's like a chemical factory."

Steve looked agitated. "You're freaking me out, man. A factory for *what?*"

There was no point in trying to soften the blow, Paul thought. He'd better just lay it on the line, like Wendy had for him. "Hey, you're not going to want to hear this any more than I did, but just like you said a moment ago, the belly fat is somewhat like an alien. It's extremely active, and manufactures all kinds of chemicals whose names I forget – chemicals that cause inflammation, increase cholesterol, increase blood pressure, wreak all kinds of havoc in the system. To put it bluntly, the chemicals it produces will kill us if we don't do something about it!"

"You're kidding me!" said Steve. "Why haven't I heard anything about this? It might have scared me into doing something sooner."

Paul shook his head. "Dr. Wendy told me it was pretty new science, but we'll be hearing all about it in the next few years. So

I did a lot of research. And it's a bummer, but it's absolutely true. That alien you're tapping away at will hasten your demise if you don't get rid of it."

Steve stopped tapping his belly and pointed at it instead. "You mean there's a *thing* in there that's out to get me?"

Paul looked Steve straight in the eye again. "Yep, as best I can understand it. But it doesn't have intent, like an alien might. You can think of it as a complex chemical factory that's polluting your insides. That's why I got rid of mine, and that's why you need to get rid of yours."

Steve straightened right up. "Yes, yes, yes. This thing has been driving me nuts for years, but I always thought it was *me*, so I gave it some slack."

"No," said Paul. "It's not 'you', exactly. It's an unfortunate addition that should never have gotten a building permit."

Steve jumped out of his chair. "Well I'm gonna tear it down. Show me what I have to do."

"OK," replied Paul with some glee. "You just say 'no'. You state your goals and you choose what silhouette you want to become."

"Oh, so we're back to the silhouettes," said Steve. "What's the deal with those?"

Paul jumped right in. "Dr. Wendy said scientists developed these figures over 20 years ago to help people recognize what weight they were. So here's the next question, Stevie. Which one would you like to be? Or, putting it another way, which one is the real you, underneath all the extra fat?"

"That's easy," said Steve. "I'd be right where you are. Number four. In fact, I like the way you said that because it's really who I am underneath it all."

Paul could see that his brother was already making sense of it. "Yes, it is simple," he quickly affirmed. "And that's who you will become if you want to. The good news is it doesn't matter how much fat you want to lose. The more you have, the longer it takes, that's all. No big deal."

"OK" said Steve. "I've chosen my silhouette. When do we get to the food part?"

"Soon enough," said Paul. "Don't you ever think about anything else? But we're not finished with this part yet. The next piece took me by surprise."

Steve jumped in. "How many surprises are you going to lay on me, Pauley?"

Paul shrugged his shoulders with his palms upturned. "Oh, just one more for the moment, so stay with me. First of all, can you see yourself getting back to number four?"

"Oh yes. I've wanted that for years," Steve exclaimed. "You're standing right in front of me and that's what I need to look like!"

Paul walked around behind his brother. "All right, so here's the harder part. Do you care enough that even if I wasn't standing here, you could see it in your mind's eye?"

Steve turned and looked at him quizzically. "I see you're serious," he said, turning away again. "So let me tell you this. I can close my eyes right now and see myself as number four."

"There you go," said Paul. "And that's where you start. You have to begin with the end in mind. So here's the final part. People get better results when they declare their intention by writing it down. Then they sign it and then tell at least two or three other people."

"Ouch," said Steve. "That just made my stomach tie in knots!"

"Sometimes people feel that way," said Paul, barely suppressing a laugh. "But if you knew that this was going to improve your chances, wouldn't you do it?" he said, composing himself. "And remember, that the knot in your stomach isn't *you*. It's the enemy at the gate."

Steve dropped his shoulders, looking uneasy. "This is really pushing my buttons, so make it simple for me."

"OK, you got it," Paul chipped in quickly. "Come on, put that dessert down. Sign off on what you are going to do and go show it to our sister and her husband!"

Steve looked perturbed. "What am I going to say?"

"Easy," replied Paul. "Just write this. 'I, Steve, commit to reducing the fat in my body from my current silhouette number seven to my real and future silhouette number four.' Now sign and date it."

Steve started scribbling quickly. "All right, I got it, I got it."

"Oh, and just one more thing," Paul added. "When you begin this, get mentally ready to receive compliments, because the weight loss happens quickly, and people will notice. I've already found that people respect anyone who is able to lose weight, because they've all tried and failed. Now get out your notepad and write this down. 'Set my goal by choosing my silhouette.'"

A note to myself

Chapter 2:
State Your Goals

Alien in the belly
The chemical factory
Where am I now?
Where do I want to go?
Make the commitment
Tell a bunch of people

Chapter Three:
Tried But Untrue

"Ouch." said Steve emerging hurriedly from the living room. "That went mostly well."

"Why 'mostly'? Did someone give you grief?" said Paul, looking up from his desk.

"Yeah, big Aunt May said it was hokey and I would never get it done," replied Steve with a smirk.

"And did you believe her?" Paul said. "She certainly knows all about weight *gain*, doesn't she?"

"Hey, I know you said I was going to get this done by learning to calibrate my food, but Aunt May's comment did wobble my confidence a bit," Steve said as he flopped despondently back into the recliner. It reminded me I'd sent away for some of those weight loss products on TV, and I wasn't successful at all."

"In fact," he went on, pointing at the muted TV on the wall, "See the ad that's on there right now? I ordered that but the food tasted like cardboard. I dropped a few pounds but put them right back on as soon as I started eating regular food."

Paul looked over at his brother. "Now why do you suppose that would be, Mr. Engineer?"

"I know, I know, it's because that's what regular food is calibrated to do, right?" responded Steve, saying ca-li-bra-ted, one syllable at a time. "Hook you back in. Well they hooked me every time."

"Got it," exclaimed Paul. "And Wendy says this is why so many people fail over and over. She told me about patients who'd tried a *dozen* different diets before, but they always ended up back where they started, sometimes even worse."

"That would be me," said Steve, tapping his forefinger on his chest.

"But here's what Wendy said," Paul continued. "There are lots of reasons most diets don't work. Some don't work because people try to diet using regular food, and it's too easy to get off track. Others are just too boring, because they have to eat the same thing meal after meal, like only cookies or shakes, so they blow the diet out of sheer rebellion."

"But the biggest reason they fail is because they go back to what they were doing before."

"Well isn't that a reasonable thing?" said Steve. "My weight is stable now. It hasn't changed for a couple of years. It's just that I'm a lot heavier than I'd like. So I figure if I just do whatever it takes, short-term, to get the weight off, then should I be able to go back to eating the way I was before and stay stable at that lower weight, right? Or, am I missing something?"

Paul leaned back, using both hands to point at his brother. "Yes, you are. And it's the most important point. It's why almost everyone gains their extra weight back."

Steve looked excited. "So you know the secret, do you? This I gotta hear."

"Think about it this way," said Paul. "You're driving along the freeway doing 70 miles an hour and you do that by pushing the gas pedal down to a particular spot and holding it there. If you push it harder, you go faster, and if you lift off you will slow down."

"OK," Steve nodded.

"So you could lift off the gas and go all the way down to 30 miles an hour, then hold the pedal in that position, and cruise along at 30 all day," Paul continued. "But what happens the moment you push the pedal back to where it was when you were doing 70 miles an hour?"

"Simple," said Steve. "You go right back to 70."

"What everyone forgets is that the human body works the same way," Paul went on. "Pushing the gas pedal is the equivalent of choosing what type and quantity of food you put in your system. Whatever you choose defines where you end up. It's really that simple. Just as you can't go 30 with the gas pedal at 70, you can't stay thin on the food that got you fat."

Steve looked a little despondent. "Does that mean I can never go back and eat whatever I want?"

"Not what you were eating before, because if you do, you'll end up in exactly the same place," replied Paul. "Didn't we just figure that out?"

"Oh man, that's kinda scary," Steve said, looking at his dessert. "I love my food so much."

"And who do you think wants you to feel that way," said Paul, looking a little smug.

Steve was getting the hang of it by now. "I know. It's the food companies, the marketing agencies and their shareholders."

"Right," said Paul. "As soon as that food gets its claws back into you, you want to eat more of it because that's how it's calibrated."

"So what am I left with? Lettuce?" Steve said, looking despondent again.

"There's lot of great food out there that won't mess you up. You just need to get the hang of it." Paul reached over and picked up a deck of playing cards from the coffee table. "Check this out," he said. "Wendy showed me the best illustration of what's going on. Once you see it, you'll never forget. Let me deal you a couple of cards."

He shuffled the deck, cut it, shuffled again and dealt Steve two cards. "Like any other card game, your objective is to choose a winning hand."

Steve picked up the cards and squinted at them. They were both clubs, a six and a nine. "OK, you need three other cards to make up your hand," said Paul. "But instead of me dealing you random cards, I'm going to turn the deck over, fan it out, and let you pick the cards you want. How does that sound?"

"Sounds like a no-brainer," said Steve with a smile on his face. He started pointing at cards as soon as Paul fanned out the deck. "I'll take the queen, king and ace of clubs." He removed them from the deck one at a time, and placed them face up beside the first two with a triumphant flourish. Slowly, he turned the remaining two face up. "There, a straight flush. Beat that!"

"It didn't take too much thought once you knew the rules, did it?" said Paul.

"Sure didn't," Steve replied. "But what on earth has this got to do with losing weight?"

"Simple," said Paul. "The first card I dealt you represents your genes; your genetic makeup. This is what you came into the world with. The second represents other things you had no choice about when you were a kid, like the food that was put on your plate."

"Seems to me the kids these days just get to eat whatever they want and it's usually junk," said Steve. "And even if they get decent food at home, they find the junk elsewhere, like at their school or the corner store. But point taken, go on. What are the three other cards?"

"Glad you asked. They represent the choices you make yourself." Paul pointed at each in turn. "Food and drink, exercise, lifestyle. They could represent lots of other things, too, but for now, we're going to say they represent food, because we make those choices every day, right?"

"Right," said Steve. "At least until you get addicted."

"All right, next question." Paul picked up Steve's cards and fanned them out. "In the card game, are you always going to pick the winning cards when you have the choice?"

"No doubt about it. Every time."

Paul pressed on. "Would you ever pick a low card?"

"Not a chance." Steve thought about it for a moment. "Unless I was already holding two of the same, but only if it made the best possible hand."

"Right," said Paul. "So you would always, without exception, choose the best possible hand."

"Yes," replied Steve. "And I can see where you're going with this."

"Exactly." Paul was enjoying seeing his brother engaged in the process. He flicked at the three cards Steve had chosen. "So in the card game of life, where these represent food, most people in this country spend their whole lives picking twos and threes: junk food, processed food, candy, soda, high fructose corn syrup and lots of others."

Steve cut in quickly. "Not just in this country, bro. I managed to mess it up a long way from here."

"I was wondering about that. What on earth were you eating?"

"I'm not crazy about the ethnic stuff as you know. But there was an American-style supermarket and I bought everything there." Steve shrugged his shoulders as he spoke. "I've been eating nothing but down-home American food and fast food when I could get it."

"No lettuce?" joked Paul. "But seriously, you weren't eating any fresh food? Produce?"

Shaking his head slowly, Steve said "It wasn't set up that way. It was what you would call 'aisle food'. He quickly straightened up in his chair. "Hey, I know what's been going on. I've been locked into that vicious cycle of poorly calibrated food you talked about. I still am."

"Right," said Paul. "Let's get back to the card game and the wrinkle I haven't told you yet. Remember we talked about how the food companies and the advertising people are always up to one trick or another?"

Paul took Steve's cards again and turned them over. "What the advertising folks do is exactly like painting the back of a card to look like the front of a card. This is how the billions of dollars get spent, making a two look like a king or whatever. And that's exactly what's happening every time every time they succeed in selling you a junk food masquerading as something good for you. Or convince you not to care. Or convince you to go for the taste and ignore the consequences."

"So people are picking the wrong stuff thinking it's the right stuff?" said Steve, looking confused again. "I've often picked the wrong stuff, but I knew full well it's the wrong stuff. I just like it."

"That's why Dr. Wendy says advertising is as much of a problem as anything else," said Paul. "The messages are so strong that people are almost having their choices made for them. Combine that with the type of food science that creates addictive tastes and textures out of cheap ingredients and people end up helpless.

The advertising 'soup' we're all swimming in around the clock is simply how the deck gets stacked in their favor."

"OK, Paul, I get all this, but here's my problem." Steve sat forward with a thoughtful look. "I just don't want to fail again and all these other diet programs I've tried, I've failed on."

"There were a lot of things you tried that turned out not to be true," Paul sympathized. "I learned that there's no magic bullet for weight loss, as some people would like you to believe. You just have to understand what to do, then do it, then keep doing it."

"The other good news is that you don't have to play from the stacked deck. I learned to pick face cards. You can too. And by the way, that's the next of the six things you need to know. Jot it down brother. Jot it down."

Tried But Untrue.

A note to myself

Chapter 3:
Tried But Untrue

Do what works
Avoid what doesn't
Keep it off
I can't stay thin eating what got me fat
Pick a winning hand
Avoid the stacked deck

Chapter Four:
Eat Calibrated Foods

People were beginning to drift aimlessly into the living room, and a couple of the younger kids started playing on the couch next to Steve. He watched them for a while and even jousted with them for a bit, but it didn't take long before he turned back to Paul with a pained yet earnest look on his face.

"So Paul," he started. "You've got my brain going, but you still haven't explained the eating part. And for me, that's pretty critical. How am I going to get this done?" He waved the notepad at Paul. "I've written down the things you said."

Enemy At The Gate.
State Your Goals.
Tried But Untrue.

"And I have to admit that Dr. Wendy's clever," he continued, "because I remember what they all mean."

"You do?" Paul responded. "So tell me."

"Hey, I've got this down," Steve said confidently. "One, they're always out to get you, so watch out; two, you've got to know where you're going so you don't end up somewhere else; and three, there are a whole lot of things out there that don't work. Did I get it?"

Paul responded, "Looks like you're on track."

Steve threw his hands up. "Well fine, but it sure seems like this would be a good time to talk about what to do. What am I going to eat?"

"OK, it's time to get into it," Paul said as he wheeled around. "Let's get away from this racket. Come on."

Paul headed into the kitchen as Steve ambled in behind. "Here," said Paul. "Pick a bar stool, any bar stool."

"You think you're funny, don't you?" jibed Steve.

"Well, didn't I get it from you?" Paul shot back. "So, pick up your pen. Here's the fourth thing Wendy told me, and you know it already. Eat calibrated foods."

"Hold it right there," Steve cut in. "You told me that's what I was doing wrong – eating food that's calibrated for the food companies."

"Yep, you're right," said Paul, pulling a bar stool away from the counter and settling himself in. "What I meant is that you should eat properly calibrated foods. Properly. Appropriately. Correctly. Ideally . . ."

"All right, smart alec," said Steve, sounding exasperated. "So what calibrated foods are you talking about? And can I get them at the corner store?"

"Not exactly," said Paul, smiling. "There *are* a handful of things there, once you've learned to do your own calibration, but it's too easy for beginners to get in big trouble. What I've learned to do these last couple of years is to calibrate my own foods because I know what those are now. I didn't before."

Paul drew a square in the air with his finger. "I shop around the outside edges of the grocery store – for vegetables, some fruit, fish, meat . . ."

"And the bakery section?" Steve interjected.

"Well not at first, because most of those foods set your system off in the wrong direction," Paul replied. "Wendy always says you have to control the food . . ."

"I got it," Steve butted in, ". . . and not let the food control you."

"Right," agreed Paul. "I broke my own rules today and ate some party food because we've got company, but I'll be right back to normal tomorrow."

Steve rubbed his hands with glee. "So celebrating is OK?"

"Sure, we all have to celebrate, that's part of life. Just not every day, which is what most of us do. People from other countries are shocked by how much food Americans stuff down every day." Paul paused for a moment. "Hey, do you remember what grandma used to say about food when we were growing up?"

"Remind me," said Steve.

"She said 'In the morning you eat like a king (or queen), at lunch you eat like a prince (or princess) and in the evening you eat like a pauper.'"

Steve nodded. "Oh yeah, I haven't heard that in 30 years. Times sure have changed. I know plenty of people who skip breakfast, have a light lunch and head home for a non-stop binge until they hit the sack."

"Well guess what? Dr. Wendy tells me that Grandma's old story has merit. Scientists have found that people who eat a hearty breakfast tend to live longer."

Steve chuckled. "Well assuming those folks don't pig out later in the day, right?"

"For sure," replied Paul. "And, a hearty breakfast is not always what people think it is."

"Paul, have you joined the food police?" said Steve mockingly.

"No, of course not," Paul retorted. Then he paused for a moment, looking thoughtful. "You know Stevie, I suppose I have, sort of, but it doesn't feel as bad as it sounds. I'm certainly way more careful than I used to be. And a lot healthier as a result."

Paul swiveled around on the bar stool and stood up beside the counter. "Here's the kind of thing I'm talking about. I went into one of those super-fancy health food supermarkets and ordered a two-egg veggie omelet from the hot counter. The cook asked me if I wanted some fried potatoes. I said 'no thanks', but he wouldn't take no for an answer."

"A muffin, then?"
"No thanks."
"Hey, it's free, you know. You're paying for it with the omelet."
"It's OK, I really just want the omelet."
"What about a bagel?"
"No thanks"
"Toast?"
"No thanks"
"Some fruit?"
"No thanks. Really, I'm fine."

"Man," Steve interrupted. "I would have taken them all."

"That's exactly the point." Paul agreed. "Everyone wants to get the most for their money. Stores like customers to feel they're offering value, and it's hard to resist when it's free. But it's not. It carries a hidden cost."

"I dunno," said Steve, patting his belly again. "It doesn't look hidden to me."

"Here's another question for you. Do actually you know how much you need to eat? In calories?"

"No idea," joked Steve. "I could tell you in platefuls, but calories, no way."

"According to Dr. Wendy, it's about 2,000 per day for a guy and 1,800 for a gal," said Paul, trying to be serious.

"I wouldn't know a calorie if it passed me on the street," said Steve.

Paul pressed on. "Next question. What mileage does your car get?"

"Ah, now that I can answer," said Steve, beaming. "20 around town and 27 on the highway."

"And how do you know that?" said Paul.

Steve was quick to reply. "I track it all the time. I keep a log in the car and every time I put in gas, I work it out. It's my engineering mind. I calculate things."

Paul grinned, knowing he was about to lower the boom. "And if you had to choose between your car and your body, which one would you keep?"

"Well, of course, the body," replied Steve, knowing he'd been nailed. "The car's not much use without it."

"Next question." Paul was on a roll. "Would you ever over-fill the tank? I mean, put 30 gallons in if it could hold only 15?"

Steve thought he had a smart answer. "Na, not a chance. The detector on the pump handle always stops it before it spills."

"Fair enough. Too bad your mouth doesn't have one of those detectors too," Paul jousted back. "So what happens if you overfill your body."

"Well, then it turns to fat, right?" Steve shot back. "That omentum again. My omentum has momentum." He furrowed his brow. "But Pauley, the annoying thing is, why doesn't it just pass through?"

"Ah, good point. I asked that same question," said Paul. "Dr. Wendy said the body is set up the way it is because we didn't always have grocery stores on every corner. There were times of plenty and times of famine all through history, as there are to this day in many countries. The body is set up to store anything that isn't used in case of a future famine."

"Oh, just like a bear does before it hibernates," Steve piped up.

"Precisely," Paul replied. "Wendy says the body is like the IRS. It keeps everything it possibly can." They both chuckled. "Every calorie you eat," he went on, "will either be used or stored, but never, ever wasted. In your case, your body used all those extra calories to make that belly."

"Well, I must have had a lot of extra calories," Steve complained. "I'm just not sure I even know how to tell how many calories are in everything. I bet that coffee I had at the airport was loaded with them."

"You're not kidding," Paul affirmed. "I don't think most people realize that some of the fancy coffees they drink on the way to work can have a third of their total calories for the day. And by then it's not even 9am."

"And that's without the muffin or the donut, right?" added Steve. "So what chance do these folks have?"

"None, unless they keep it under control, which most don't because it becomes habitual. That's the way the food companies like it."

"Pauley, you're driving me nuts," Steve said, putting his head in his hands. "The more I think about this the more it scares me. How can I possibly go out and keep choosing the right things when everything's set up to derail me."

"Don't worry," said Paul. "You're about to find out."

"Before I do, where's that wrongly calibrated dessert I was working on?" said Steve, brightening up. "I must have left it in the other room." He started to get up but Paul stopped him.

"Hang on a minute. There's no shortage of dessert today." Paul walked over to the refrigerator, pulled out a bowl and slid it along the counter to Steve. "Give this a shot," he said, tossing him a spoon.

"OK, you made me do it," said Steve. "This looks yummy – what is it? Chocolate pudding? Fruit? Some vanilla too?"

Paul nodded and watched with a smile as Steve started eating. "Dang, this is tasty," he said, speaking as he ate. "Too bad they can't make 'properly calibrated' food taste like this."

"Well, Steve, that's where you'd be wrong." Paul was wearing a triumphant grin. "They can, and they did. That's a 'properly calibrated' dessert."

"Yowza! I could eat this all day long." Steve looked up between bites. "So what's the difference between this and a regular dessert? I can't *taste* any difference."

Paul was happy to explain. "The big thing is it's chock full of protein, as much as in a couple of eggs, but there are almost no carbs, moderate fat levels, low calories and some fiber."

"And this is how you lost weight? By eating stuff like this?" asked Steve.

"You're darn right. Every two or three hours." Paul replied.

Steve looked astonished. He did some quick mental arithmetic. "You ate, what, six times a day and you lost weight?"

"Yep, sometimes seven." Paul loved explaining this part to people, and it just made it better that this time it was for his dear brother. "The fat starts to disappear as soon as you calibrate your food so your body will do that. Remember how we talked about the body's calibration being fixed, so you have to adjust the fuel according to what you want it to do?"

"Yes, I think I have that one down pat," said Steve as he finished up his dessert and leaned over the counter to put the bowl in the sink. "Now I just have to do it. And if it's all like *that* I can do it easily."

Paul walked back behind the counter and started to rinse the bowl. "One thing I realized at Dr. Wendy's was that I was fighting with myself. Part of me wanted to lose weight, but another part of me didn't want to change a thing . . ."

"Must have been your omentum," quipped Steve. "So how did you get over that?"

"It happened in Dr. Wendy's office that first visit . . ."

- - - - - -

Paul pulled the list out of his pocket and handed it to Wendy. "I've been battling myself over the issues I wrote there," he said. "I know myself well enough to know that if any one of them is missing, it's going to make it more difficult for me to succeed. Can you solve this for me?"

Wendy scanned the list quickly then looked at Paul over the top of her glasses. "So aside from wanting it to work, you want the food to be varied, convenient, and easy to prepare because you don't like cooking. You want it to be simple, and something your family can use too. You don't want to starve yourself, in fact you don't want to feel hungry at all. And on top of all that you want it to be tasty. Oh, and you don't want it to break the bank. Did I get that right?"

"That would be precisely correct," Paul replied, a little sheepishly.

"Well, you're not the only one who feels that way," she replied. "The food companies and advertisers have worked for decades getting people programmed to depend on taste and convenience."

"Paul, I heard that question so often I figured I'd better find an approach that would really work for people. Everyone is so accustomed to having everything they need at their fingertips that if they don't have properly calibrated foods right in front of them they'll tend to go astray."

"So guess what?" She got up and motioned for Paul to follow. "You'll be doing most of your shopping here for the next few months."

They walked down through the waiting room and into a door on the other side. "Here you are," said Wendy. "Nutritionally designed foods calibrated for weight loss."

"Wow", said Paul, gazing at shelves filled with boxes of food. "I think I should be able to find something here."

Wendy walked around the room, picking out boxes and handing them to Paul. "Some of these, like the protein bars, are ready to eat," she said. "Others just need water added, some cold, some hot. There's oatmeal, puddings, bars, shakes, soups. You can dress the soups up with some frozen vegetables if you like. Do you think this could work for you?"

"It sure looks like it. Do you provide me with some kind of plan, so I know what to eat at what time of day?" Paul asked as he examined the boxes.

"I could, but here's the trick." Wendy turned some of the boxes over and showed Paul the labels. "They're all the same, so you can switch them around. Everything has 15 grams of protein, 80-130 calories each, very few carbs and moderate fat. Some have vitamins too. And because the protein satisfies the body in a way that all the carbs in regular food don't, you won't get hungry for at least a couple of hours."

Paul was starting to feel confident about his weight issues for the first time. "Cool, so I eat one of these every two hours, and it doesn't matter which one?"

"That's right," she said.

"I have to tell you I'm pretty excited," said Paul, holding up the boxes. "I had no idea you could even get these. Why aren't they in stores?"

"Simple economics," Wendy shrugged. "Protein is a much more expensive ingredient than carbs, and the price won't be driven down until more people demand foods that are calibrated this way."

"So," she continued, "You eat one of these every two to three hours, and one regular meal a day that has only protein and vegetables: fish, chicken, lean meat, soy protein, whatever you

prefer. I'll give you a list of all the foods you can use."
Paul smiled approvingly. "And it's that simple?"

"It's that simple."

"Does this work for everybody?" said Paul as they headed back
out of the room. "I was thinking about my wife, Meg."

"Oh yes," replied Wendy, "In fact, two-thirds of my patients
who have done this are women. They drop weight a *little* slower
than men because their metabolism is more complex, but look
at Caroline's picture on the wall there. She dropped 34 pounds
in three months. Pretty good, huh?"

"Wow, pretty spectacular. It happens that fast?" said Paul, a little
surprised. "Is that safe?"

"Yes, very safe, "said Wendy. "This type of program has been
studied extensively, and is even included in guidelines by the
National Institutes of Health for managing obesity. Plus, the
rapid weight loss does wonders for people's confidence and
keeps them on track."

- - - - - -

"So, Steve, here it is," said Paul, opening the pantry door.
"Everything I need is right here, and I take it wherever I go."

Steve jumped off his bar stool and darted into the pantry.
He started muttering half to himself and half to Paul, while
feverishly grabbing boxes. "This is OK, mmm chocolate, I could
eat this, mediterranean tomato soup, looks tasty, crunchy snacks,
those'll keep me off the chips . . ." He came back out of the

pantry clutching a pile of boxes. "Pauley, if I started this right now, how far do you think I'd get in the month I'm here?"

"Far enough that you'll want me to keep shipping them to you." Paul slapped him on the back. "Come on. Let's go entertain the guests . . ."

A note to myself

Chapter 4:
Eat Calibrated Foods

Choose my food
Shop the perimeter
Learn to say no
Know my body's "mileage"
Start the day right
Buy properly calibrated foods until
I can learn to calibrate my own

Chapter Five:
Enhance Your Success

Wendy stepped out of the product room just in time to see Paul and Steve walk into the office.

"Hey Paul," she said as she walked towards them. "So you've brought me the Incredible Shrinking Man? You guys *do* look alike."

Steve smiled and held out his hand. "Hi Doc, pleased to meet you. I've heard a lot about you. In fact, it feels like I've already had a bunch of appointments with you."

"Well, Paul's become a good spokesman for me, and in this office we always say we like to see less of people more often," she quipped. "Let's go on back." Wendy turned and headed for the corridor with the brothers in tow.

"Steve's been running around all over the place, with so many people to see," said Paul. "He's heading back out of the country tomorrow, so I'm glad you were able to fit him in."

"That's a happy thing for me, too," Wendy replied as she made her way behind the desk. "Go ahead and pull the chairs up and we'll chat. Now Steve, this is your appointment, so is it OK for Paul to be here?"

"Oh yeah, we can let him stick around, don't you think?" said Steve, nodding towards his brother.

"Great. Works for me if it works for you." Wendy picked up her clipboard and began writing. "So, I know Paul's been getting you the food from our program, and you've been on it for how long now?"

"Just less than a month," Steve replied. "I was over here for my sister's wedding, so I got that feast out of the way before I started."

"Good plan. And how much weight have you lost?" said Wendy.

"Fourteen pounds," Steve exclaimed. "Seven in the first week, then three a week after that."

"Yes, that's not unusual the first week. People tend to lose a lot of water they've been holding on to, then it levels out. Have you been hungry at all?" she asked.

"Not at all," he responded. "In fact, sometimes I have to remind myself it's time to eat. I've put an alarm on my computer, since I spend so much time in front of it." Steve paused for a moment. "The first two or three days were odd. It was as though my body was resisting, and I kept wanting things I couldn't have, but since day four I don't even care any more."

Wendy looked up from her notes. "And you know why that is?"

"Paul told me the body gets into patterns, and when you try to change them it resists. Truthfully I thought it would take longer than it did."

"It's very fast for most people," Wendy confirmed. "And how have you been feeling since then?"

"I just can't believe how much energy I have. I thought this whole thing might be a battle, but I just *had* to do it after seeing mister skinny over there," he responded. "And I'm not kidding, I don't get tired at all during the day. I used to fall asleep after lunch, but not any more."

"Excellent, it sounds like you're right on track. How have the folks around you reacted?"

"Funny you should ask that. When I first got here I felt terrible, and although people were polite, except *him* . . ." Steve pointed at Paul, "I knew they were discussing my size, because I'd never been that big. But now that they're seeing such dramatic results, I get nothing but compliments. My face visibly thinned almost right away, and now my body's following."

"Great," said Wendy. "Just make sure you keep drinking enough water between meals. Are you taking the custom supplements Paul ordered for you? We provide them to almost every patient."

"You mean these?" Steve pulled out a little packet of capsules from his shirt pocket. "Yeah I think it's neat that they're made for me. Haven't missed a day, and I think they're really helping too. I notice my hair is thicker and my nails don't crack so easily. What role do those play in the program?"

"A very important one." Wendy got up and walked over to the wall. Come over and take a look at this. Paul's seen it before."

"Yeah," Paul piped up from his chair. "It's my street map."

"Looks more like an engineering schematic to me," suggested Steve.

"You're not far off," said Wendy, pointing to a series of lines in the middle of the chart. "These all depict chains of chemical reactions in the body, where one substance gets made into another. For example, this whole section relates to energy production, and this one over here to detoxification. Notice anything?"

Steve laughed. "Only a bunch of names I don't recognize."

She pointed at a tiny piece of writing. "What about these?"

"Oh, he said," peering closer. "That's Mg, magnesium, and that says B-6, a B-vitamin. There's calcium. OK, I see what you're saying now."

"Right. Your entire body needs vitamins, minerals and other compounds to work properly," Wendy explained. "We need macronutrients, big compounds like protein, fat and carbs, but we also need the micronutrients. That's where your supplements come in. They're designed to match your own metabolism."

"Don't people say you get all you need from your food?" asked Steve.

Wendy shook her head. "Not a chance, at least not any more. You would have to have perfect conditions and eat a perfect diet grown on perfect soil. But the problem is that even when people get good nutrition from their food, there are too many other things stripping it out again, like pollution and stress, to name only two."

"That's a sobering picture," said Steve. "I really didn't know it was that bad. But I will acknowledge, I didn't even know until a few weeks ago that I could even feel this good any more. I thought it had gone and wasn't coming back."

"It's amazing what the body will do when given the right fuel," said Wendy. "And the micronutrients and water work well together during weight loss to help move chemicals out of your body."

"What chemicals?" said Steve, a little startled. "I didn't know I had chemicals on board."

"People are continually exposed to all kinds of chemicals. They're in the environment, fumes, drugs, furniture, homes, all kinds of places," said Wendy. "And they're mostly fat-soluble, so as fat gets stored in your body, many of these are stored with it. Exactly how much depends on what you've been exposed to, but as you lose weight and your fat breaks down, you can feel pretty funky unless your system is well primed to get them out of there."

"Wow," said Steve. "I learn something new every day. And hey, talking of chemicals, will this help me get off my cholesterol drug?"

"Oh, don't get me started on cholesterol," Wendy said, rolling her eyes back in her head: "That's one of the biggest misinformation campaigns in history. Cholesterol is not the villain it's made out to be. The problems associated with it are really more to do with inflammation and other factors. Look up 'cholesterol skeptics' online and you'll see the other side of the story. But yes, we see may people whose cholesterol and triglycerides improve and some even normalize."

"Cool," said Steve.

Wendy walked back over to her desk and glanced at Paul. "Looks like you're getting your body double back," she said, nodding her head in Steve's direction. He was still tracing lines on the chart. "Hey, Steve, how much more weight do you want to lose?"

"Oh, I think it's 50-something pounds. It'll take me a few months at this rate," he said as he returned to his seat.

"Well do you want to kick it up a notch?" Wendy asked.

"Not if I have to starve," he said. "I like my new food, and Paul's going to ship it out to me."

"No, this is an eating program, not a starving program," said Wendy. "I'm talking about exercise. Proper nutrition is by far the biggest part of weight loss, but getting some exercise really ups the ante."

"I haven't felt much like exercise these last few years, but now my energy is up again, I suppose it's a possibility," he replied. "What did you have in mind?"

"Most people just start out walking, unless they want to get fancier," Wendy suggested. "To start with, just get a pedometer and do a few thousand steps a day. Getting it up to ten thousand daily is great."

"Phew, ten thousand sounds like a lot," replied Steve, making breathless sounds.

"You'll be amazed as how fast it adds up when you do little things like park your car further away from the store, or take the stairs at the office," Wendy reassured him, "And the right pace to walk at when you're doing it for exercise is where you can still have a conversation – a slightly breathless one. That tells you you're in the right zone."

"Yes doctor," said Steve in a deliberately formal tone. "Whatever you say."

"There's just one more thing that'll put the icing on the cake," Wendy grinned, "One you might not expect."

"Oh, I get to have a cocktail?" joked Steve.

"Actually, better than that," she said. "It's important to get enough sleep while you're losing weight. I know you have all this newfound boundless energy, but get at least 8 hours, preferably 9, but never less than 7 every single night."

"Well, there's good news there, doc," Steve replied. "I used to have really bad sleep apnea, but it's already started to diminish. And by the way, my blood pressure has started to drop too."

"Great – you're definitely on track," said Wendy. "And it just gets better from here. These things we've been talking about, water, supplements, exercise and sleep, I call 'nature's helpers'. They just help the weight loss process along and enhance your results. You'll see." She paused for a moment, the looked up again. "Hey, has Paul had you writing down the six things?"

"Sure has," replied Steve, "We're at number 4."

"It's time to write another one, so write 'Enhance Your Success'," she said. "Because that's what's about to happen . . ."

A note to myself

Chapter 5:
Enhance Your Success

Take custom supplements
Stay hydrated
Take a walk
Move my body

Chapter Six:
Mastering Your Mind

Paul eased the car out of the driveway, and set off down the street at a snail's pace.

"Step on it, bro," Steve encouraged him. "I need all the time I can get. We need to be getting the gas pedal to 70 as soon as we can, not 30."

"Oh yeah, right." Paul picked up the pace a bit as they headed towards the freeway. He realized he'd unconsciously been going as slowly as he could because these were his few remaining minutes with his brother. Steve was heading back out of the country. "I can't believe how fast this month has flown by. It seems like you just got here."

"Feels that way to me, too." Steve paused for a moment. "But at the same time I feel like a totally different guy."

"Well you are. And in such a short time." It was like watching my own process all over again. "Hey," Paul asked, "Can you still recall how you felt when you stepped out of that cab."

"You mean how it felt to be fat?" said Steve. "You're forgetting I still am. But yes, I remember how nervous I was, and I'd taken the cab so you wouldn't walk right past me at the airport. I also felt physically uncomfortable … I have for years now. And I can also tell you I will never forget that feeling. I'm never going back."

Steve was emphatic as he continued. "I'm finally on my way, I have something that works, and as I begin introducing new foods, I know I always have something to fall back on. So I'm taking this all the way down to 172 pounds." He laughed. "Not to be competitive, of course."

"Of course not," exclaimed Paul, "But if you're going to be competitive about anything, this would be a good thing to pick. Remember too, that you've got a few prescriptions to get off too. That's part of the competition."

"If you did, I will," Steve shot back. "And by then I'll be able to give you a good drubbing on the basketball court." He turned and pointed out the passenger window at the outdoor court they virtually lived in as kids. "I thought someone would have built something on there by now."

"Not yet," Paul replied, "But I'm sure it's just a matter of time. Hey, I know you're doing fine here, but how do you think you're going to do on your own?"

"I gotta tell you, Pauley, a month in and I have absolutely no interest in doing anything else. Everything's better. Not just my weight, but also my attitude, my confidence. I'm even thinking better," Steve said confidently.

"Well that would be a first," jibed Paul. "Never saw that before."

"Ha, ha," Steve retorted. "No, I'm very clear already. This is a permanent thing for me. I've struggled with my weight for years, and now I know why. I understand calibration and I'm going to pay as much attention to me as I do to my car from now on. I'm not getting ensnared again in the trap of mis-calibrated foods."

Steve's face brightened. "And I'm going to get to shop in my closet for at least a few months. I never threw out any of those smaller clothes after the last thirty pounds of weight gain, because I always figured I would somehow get it handled and I would need them again. Now I do."

"I did the exactly the same thing," said Paul with a chuckle. "Her ladyship kept wanting to take them to the thrift store, and I wouldn't let her – though by the time I got real skinny, even *they* were hanging on me like a tent."

"Well look at this," said Steve, tugging at his belt. "I'm already down one, almost two holes on my belt."

"Way to go, bro," Paul acknowledged with a smile. Then his expression got serious. "So do you think you can keep your mindset firm once you get back into work, social life and events without getting swept up in it all? It can get tough, as I found."

"Not a chance!" replied Steve. "If the food hadn't been good, I might have had trouble, but with my precious boxes always at hand, plus what I've learned hanging out with you for a month, I think I'll be just fine. In fact, I've gotten to like all the different vegetables, and eating smaller portions of lean meat. I'm sure my stomach has gotten smaller, as I just can't eat as much as I used to. I get full much sooner."

"Well you also learned to eat slower," said Paul, "And for most people that's a big lesson. Everyone's always in a rush and they eat so fast their brain doesn't have time to register it."

"I remember you saying that it takes 15-20 minutes for the brain to catch up with the stomach, and people can eat so much in that time that when the brain finally recognizes it, they're completely stuffed." A grin spread across Steve's face. "Just like when I got to your house that first day. I wouldn't do that now."

"All right, I'm hearing you're up for the fight. So now there's just one more thing I want to let you know," said Paul, as he signaled to turn off for the airport.

"There's more? I thought I was pretty well set," Steve replied. "What have you got?"

"Look there on the back seat," Paul said, pointing behind him. "Pick up that book with the yellow cover."

Steve stretched back and retrieved it. "OK, I got it. 'Break Through Your Set Point'."

"It's by Dr. George Blackburn," Paul continued. "He's a Harvard professor who's been studying obesity for decades. What he's found is that people who have been heavy for a while tend to drop their weight in stages."

"Interesting. Why is that?" Steve was intrigued.

"The body has what's called a Set Point, and it acts like a 'weight thermostat'. I'm sure you've seen actors who pack on weight for a movie then take it off again, or maybe the opposite – they get real skinny, then normalize again," said Paul.

"Yeah, they always made me jealous," said Steve. "I'd wonder how they could do that so easily, when I had such a hard time. I figured they must have personal trainers."

"Well I'm sure they do, but the point is they gained or lost the weight for only a month or two, so their body went right back to its set point."

"So it's a time thing?" asked Steve.

"Seems to be. If you stay at a particular weight for about 6 months, your set point will re-set to *that* weight, not the one you had before."

Steve looked like he had it figured out. "So that's why people boomerang back when they quit their diet?" he suggested.

"Yes, and Wendy says it's like drawing back a bow string," Paul went on, "The further you get away from your set point, the greater the pressure for it to return."

"So what do you about that?" said Steve, looking perplexed. "How do you reset it?"

"Turns out it's simple," Paul explained. "You drop some weight, hold it there for long enough to let your set point reset *to a lower weight* then start back down."

"And how far can people go at a time?" Steve asked.

"Dr. Wendy always talks about how everyone's different, and some people can go a lot further than others, depending on their metabolism and their personal discipline," said Paul. "Dr. Blackburn says it's about 10% on average. After that, the body rebels more. But some people lose a lot more before they stick."

"What do you mean stick? When they stop losing weight?" said Steve.

"Right. As people lose weight, they'll often reach a plateau. Some are short, some are longer," said Paul. "When my weight was coming down, it just fell off for quite a while, then there were a couple of periods when it didn't change at all."

"So what did you do?" said Steve.

"I just stayed with the program and, about a week later, I started back down," replied Paul. "But then I hit 190, and it wouldn't budge at all, for weeks."

"That must have made you nervous," said Steve, "But obviously you got past it."

"It was driving me nuts, because I was about 15% down at that point with 15 pounds to go," Paul recalled. "Then I remembered I'd been at that weight for years, just like you were. So I figured maybe the body had some kind of memory about being that weight before, and when I told Dr. Wendy she gave me that book. It all made sense when I read it."

"Wow," said Steve. "I wonder how many people give up because they don't know that one piece of information."

"I can't even imagine how big that number is," said Paul. "But now you know, so you won't be one of them. Take the book with you. I have another copy." He dodged around two airport shuttles, and headed for the terminal ramp.

"Just one thing, Pauley," Steve piped up, retrieving his crumpled piece of notepaper from his pocket. "What's the sixth thing I need to know?"

"Glad you asked. It's just what we've been talking about on the drive," Paul replied. "Mastering Your Mind. It's all about not being fooled. Staying true to your goals, not being swayed by friends, co-workers, food companies, advertising, your own mental tricks, or even your set point."

As Steve wrote, he suddenly jerked his head back. "Hey Paul, did you notice this?"

Paul saw a car leaving a curbside spot and quickly nipped into it. "Notice what?"

"When I write all these things down, look at what they say. Look at the first letters."

Enemy at the Gate.
State Your Goals.
Tried But Untrue.
Eat Calibrated Foods.
Enhance Your Success.
Mastering Your Mind.

"How cool is that?" Steve looked delighted. "I was going to call this the Silhouette Solution for Myself, but now I can call it . . ." He scribbled for a moment, then showed it to Paul.

"The Silhouette Solution for My Self Esteem."

"That, Pauley, is going on my bathroom wall," Steve exclaimed, brandishing the paper. "Do you think Wendy did that intentionally? Or is it just a coincidence?"

Paul looked at him with a quizzical smile. "I'll let you figure that one out for yourself."

A note to myself

Chapter 6:
Mastering Your Mind

Never forget
Stay with the program
Eat s-l-o-w-l-y
Take it in stages
Reset my set point
Don't get talked out of it

Epilogue

It turned out to be barely a year before Steve returned. He'd met and got engaged to Tess, an executive assistant who'd been transferred to his office. Best of all, the company had offered them both a transfer to the US. He was finally coming home.

He'd made great progress, too, reaching his goal of 172 pounds, give or take two or three on any given day. Just as Paul had suggested, the first 35 or so went quickly, then he stabilized for a month or so, before dropping the remainder in round two. He was proud that he'd never strayed from the program. Well, not in the big picture, anyway. Yes, there had been the occasional party, the company event, and plenty of other temptation. But even as he relished the occasional treat, he found he'd lost interest in much of what he ate before. He just felt too good. A couple of times when he overdid it, he felt some of the old sluggishness come back, even though he hadn't gained a pound. He still had a blast at parties, but simply watched what he put on his plate. Sometimes he'd have a protein snack just before he arrived, so he'd approach the table already feeling satisfied.

His regular doctor had praised his progress, and taken him off his blood pressure and cholesterol medications when he no longer needed them. "It would make my job a lot easier if everyone did what you've just done," his doctor had said.

Best of all, his weight loss had done wonders for his self confidence. Having lightness in his step made him feel like a king, and he noticed that others reacted to him differently. It was that breezy confidence that had attracted Tess. They walked and talked together every day they could. They'd even joined a gym together.

Everything had just started flowing better. Steve attributed it to him being in control of his food, rather than his food controlling him. He began to notice when foods he experimented with caused him to feel strange, or create cravings for more. He avoided those as soon as he identified them. And now he was going to be palling around with his brother again. How great was that?

- - - - - -

Paul strode out the house and downstairs into the yard where Steve and Tess were relaxing in lawn chairs. Tess looked up with a startled expression. "I have no idea how long it's going to take me to get used to this," she said. "Every time I see you I think you're Steve." Tess grabbed Steve's arm.

"You'll get the hang of it," replied Paul. "It takes only a day or two. We may look identical, and have some similar mannerisms that we picked up together as we grew, but our personalities are quite different."

"Well just don't go playing any tricks on me," said Tess, glowering playfully and wagging her finger at him.

"No need to worry. Girlfriends, spouses and fiancés get special dispensation," Paul replied, "But bosses don't . . ." he added with glee. "Are you ready, Steve-O?"

"I'm on it," said Steve as he jumped out of this chair. They both trotted up the stairs into the house. "Come on, Tess, you're in this one too."

"Oh, what have I got myself into now?" she said with weary resignation as she followed the pranksters into the house.

A minute later Paul and Steve emerged from Paul's bedroom, grinning from ear to ear. They'd both donned identical clothing: khaki pants, a dark blue dress shirt and brown loafers. Tess' heart skipped a beat. "Which was her Steve?" Then she spotted the little mole on his neck, and breathed an audible sigh of relief.

"That's really wild," she said, feeling she had to be a good sport with her future brother-in-law. "So what's the ruse?"

"Oh, this one's easy, just to get you into the swing of it," said Paul with a grin. "All I want you guys to do is what comes naturally. Just step out to the side porch, take a seat on the couch, and well, be affectionate."

"Oh, I see what you're up to, you rascals," said Tess, "But won't the neighbors have a fit if they think it's you?"

"Naaaa, they're all in on it. And they'll all be over tonight anyway." Paul explained the prank. "My boss, Jim, the news editor, is going to be arriving in a few minutes. He just called to say he's on his way. He knows Meg pretty well, so I can't wait to see the look on his face when he sees you guys canoodling on the porch." Paul giggled. "I'll be watching from behind the screen door."

It wasn't even a minute later that Jim's car drove up. He pulled into the front driveway and clambered out holding some flowers for Meg and a bottle of wine for Paul. He straightened up, rearranged the gifts and walked around, as he always did, to the side door.

Steve and Tess were curled up together on the couch, pecking each other on the cheek. As soon as Jim approached below, Steve spoke up. "Hey Jim, what you got there?" Jim was watching the steps as he came up on to the porch. "A decent bottle of red for you, Paul" he began, "And some flowers for Mmmm . . ." He tailed off as the pair came into full view. His jaw dropped.

"Eh . . . eh . . . flowers . . ." Jim stammered, "For . . . eh . . . the . . . um . . . house . . . er . . ." He thought to himself "What on earth do I do here? Are the kids here? Do they know? Where's Meg?"

Paul couldn't stand it any longer. He came bursting through the screen door, with Meg right behind him. "Hey Jim, I see you met my brother!" Jim did a double-take, then twice, then three times. "Good grief," he said, "You never told me you guys were twins." He handed the wine to Paul and the flowers to Meg. "Of course not," said Paul. "Why spoil the fun."

"You don't deserve that bottle. I just about had a heart attack," Jim continued, pretending he was clutching his chest and taking a few deep breaths. "But Meg, you absolutely deserve those flowers for living with such a scoundrel."

"And you," he said, turning to Steve. "Must be the famous, and now infamous, Steve." Steve stood up and shook his hand. "I'm delighted to meet you and I'm glad you're such a good sport. This is my fiancé, Tess. Come on in and let's pour you a drink. You deserve it after that!"

Everyone filed into the house, with Paul and Steve taking up the rear. Just as they approached the screen door, they turned and high-fived. "We're back!" said Paul. "Yeah, we sure are," said Steve, patting his brother on the back. "Life is good."